I0420842

Book 1

Paleo Diet : A quick beginner guide

Book 2

Essential oils : a quick beginner guide

By Rick Paul

Book 1

Paleo Diet

A quick beginner guide

By Rick Paul

Table of Contents

Introduction

I want to thank you and congratulate you for downloading the book, Paleo Diet.

This book contains proven steps and strategies about Paleo diet. This book is an excellent guide for people who want to know everything there is to know about the Paleo Diet. This Book is the Ultimate Guidelines for a beginner.

The Paleo diet is a low carb diet, with a high amount of protein and a lot of vegetables. This diet is sometimes referred to as the "Caveman Diet" because it is basically anything that was eaten by a caveman. This diet is so effective because it forces your body to burn fats for energy, instead of glucose from carbs.

If your goal is to lose weight, keep it off, and increase energy levels, you need to eat all natural, non processed foods like the caveman did. The caveman didn't have the technology to grow grains or make dairy products, so why would we eat them?.Adapting the caveman diet will not only help you live a healthy and fulfilling life but you will also be able to cut fat and look the way you've always wanted.

This book will provide all information needed to implement the Paleo Diet in your life.I will discuss about the Paleo,the benefits of Paleo,What you can eat when on a Paleo diet, **What Food Should You Avoid.**I will help you implement the Paleo Diet.

You will get exact and reliable information in regards to the topic and issue covered. The book is sold with the information that the publisher is not necessary to render accounting, officially acceptable, or otherwise, professional services. If information is necessary, legal or acceptable, an experienced individual in the profession should be ordered.

Thanks again for downloading this book, I hope you enjoy it!

Chapter 1   What is paleo ?

The Paleo diet is a very healthy way that you can eat because it is the one kind of food approach that works with your genetics to help you to stay slim, strong and active. Studies in biology, biochemistry, Ophthalmology, Dermatology, and many other specialties have determined that it is our new nutrition, which is full of refined food, unhealthy fats and sugar, that is at the source of progressive diseases, such as obesity, malignancy, diabetes, heart disease, and many others.

The Paleolithic food plan is a new, healthy plan that is based on the food consumed in Paleolithic times. It is based on several key ideas, including: 1. Social heredities have barely improved since the beginning of agriculture, which was about fifty thousand years back at the end of the Paleolithic age; 2. The new persons adjust to the food or diets of the Paleolithic time and; 3. It is probable for new science to determine what such a food plan consisted of.

The people who are familiar with the Paleo diet say that the modern people who exist on ordinary food, the same types believed to be consumed by Paleolithic hunter-gatherers, are mainly free from disease and have found that eating Paleolithic food has shown better health results when compared to other largely-recommended food plans.

The Paleo Diet Method

The Paleo food, which is the genuine term for food in the Paleolithic Diet method, consists of the types of food contained in the diet that the Paleolithic man would have had in prehistoric years.

There's no question that, as time has progressed onwards, knowledge and cooking procedures have significantly improved since the age of our forefathers. They would have to actually go out and search in the world for the foods for their diets. Today, we simply take a quick trip to the grocery store, where we're met with a large selection of a variety of foods that have been properly treated and prepared to eat.

The problem with this is that, while these changes have happened, we've polluted the nutrition of our regular food and are missing out on the essential elements in our food that nature intended for us to have. We've added to the convenience of food, but this has happened at the cost of nutrition.

The idea of the Paleolithic food is to go back to the natural food of prehistoric times. When accepting this dieting method, you choose to forgo all of the new types of foods that you find at the supermarket and instead focus on a diet that is natural and balanced. Basically, if it was accessible thousands of years ago, it's beneficial to have in a meal that you are planning.

Purpose of the Paleo Diet

The Paleo diet is created with the knowledge that people's figures used to be developed through the largely dependable food bases that were accessible to prehistoric collectors. Over time, the body adjusted to this diet and responded to it optimally. Preservatives and other cultivated products were presented comparatively recently in man's history, and are detrimental to the body because they are not as nutritionally valuable as the traditional foods of the Paleolithic age.

Chapter 2   The benefits of a Paleo diet

One of the mistaken beliefs about the Paleo diet is that it's focused on proteins with fat. Combine that with the improved health and increased nutrient absorption that happens through the avoidance of irritating grains and legumes, and you get a very balanced diet. You will be astonished that anyone can have all of the compulsory nutrients that are found in animal, seafood and plant created diets. Here you can see 10 Paleo diet benefits.

10 Paleo diet benefits

1. Well-developed Brain

One of the best bases of protein and fat recommended by the Paleo diet originates from icy water fish; preferably wild-caught salmon. Other bases of omega 3 fatty acids are found in pasture-raised herbs and seed.

2. Develop all Essential Vitamins & Minerals

The Paleo nutrition recommends consumption of multicolored food. Root vegetables are a great part of the diet and it's able to offer a variability of vegetables, contingent on the seasons.

The different types of vegetarians are in need of the nutrients they include! By eating the colorful foods, you confirm that you are getting all of your vitamins.

3. Good Digestion and Absorption

The Paleo Diet proposes the consumption of foods that you've acquired the skill to digest rapidly over thousands of ages. There are no questions whether or not you might bear starch or grass-fed complaints. Your ancestors lived and prospered off these diets.

4. A Smaller amount Allergies

The Paleo Diet suggests that you avoid foods that are well-known to be allergy-inducing in some societies. Some persons are incapable of processing seeds and dairy, which is why the Paleo Diet strongly suggests you limit these diets to a minimum every month.

Persons often gather that the Paleo Diet doesn't have whole grains. The reality is just that grains are not the greatest foods for energy, so we avoid them most of the time, but not continuously. If you are an athlete, you may need to consume a single cup of oats before you compete.

5. Decrease Infection

Studies propose that inflammation may be an important factor for heart disease. What you should know about the Paleo Diet is that a lot of the foods have anti-inflammatory agents so you will be reducing your danger.

The greater focus on omega 3 fatty acids is one of the benefits of those foods is that they are anti-inflammatory.

6. Extra Energy

Ever wonder why energy juices have become so standard in the last decade? It's because everybody's food sucks!

A classic American mealtime consists of a honey, coffee coupled with a muffin or bagel with cream cheese. Not only does this eventually lead to two kinds of diabetes and insulin opposition, but also it won't even keep you satiated. With the Paleo Diet, you intentionally select the correct foods all the time.

7. Weight Loss

The Paleo Diet is a low-carb diet by design. Just removing preserved nutrients radically decreases your carb consumption and results in weight loss.By avoiding carbs, you will evade an unwelcome fat increase, which is often produced by these extra carbs.

8. Decrease Danger of Disease

The Paleo Diet's main focus is to escape diets that can potentially harm your health. The Paleo diet makes it easy to avoid bad foods by giving you a simple blueprint; only eat what a caveman would be able to eat.

When this is followed, it will ensure that you eat whole foods, and limit your danger for infection by escaping the foods recognized to originate them.

9. Shrink Person's Fat Cells

Most people don't fully realize that fat cells shrink and increase based on your food. A slim person does not have less fat cell, they just have smaller cells. A way to make your fat cells smaller is to select good fats and limit your carb eating. All elements the Paleo Diet proposes. Good fats are collected within your chambers and are readily accessible for energy when someone is insulin deficient.

10. Detox Effects

When you stop consuming things that sabotage your health, such as caffeine, refined sugar, trans fats, gluten, and more, you are giving your body a break. You'll be purging your body of all the built-up toxic foods. We call this a detox. Many Paleo Dieters report that they feel lighter and more focused after just a couple of weeks. After you've had your detox, your cheat meal won't have the same satisfying effect as when you were addicted. In fact, you'll experience negative side effects immediately when you have your cheat meal. You'll suffer from diarrhea, headaches and instant bloating. This will help you to be less likely to implement cheat meals and allow you to cut out processed foods for good.

Chapter 3 What you can eat when on a Paleo diet

Many people get confused when I say that eating fat is very healthy for you. Some cannot even accept the fact that this is true. But the truth is, eating fats is very healthy for you. It has several benefits like improving bones, liver health, healthy lungs, immune system, and promoting a healthy brain. Here you can see some Paleo diet food list.

Paleo Diet Food List

Meat

Goat, sheep, horse, wild boar, pork, rabbit, lamb, beef, bison.

Game meat

Bear, moose, woodcock, elk, duck, rabbit, reindeer, wild turkey, deer, pheasant.

Fish

Salmon, trout, bass, sole, haddock, turbot, tilapia, cod, flatfish, grouper, mackerel, anchovy, tuna, walleye, halibut.

Fats

avocado oil, olive oil, avocados, coconut oil, clarified butter (ghee), lard, tallow, butter, duck fat, veal fat, lamb fat, fatty fishes, nut butters, nut oils (walnut, macadamia), milk coconut.

Paleo Diet Seafood

Down in New Orleans and want to have a gumbo? With the Paleo diet, change it out for shrimp. Want to enjoy a meal at the Red Lobster? Check out the loads of alternative seafood you can enjoy on the paleo diet.

Crab, Crawfish, Crayfish, Clams, Shrimp, Lobster, Scallops, Oysters, Mushrooms, Button mushroom, Portobello, Chanterelle, Crimini,

Paleo Diet Root vegetable

The Paleo Diet is comprised of many root vegetables. Almost all vegetables are considered in the Paleo diet as being healthy, but you still need to be aware of the starch content. Root vegetables with the maximum starch content – such as potatoes and jams - are likely to have a lower nutritional value, depending on the quantity of starches and sugars they have. Although they are not good for you, they're not completely off-limits. The following chart shows some of the accepted Paleo Diet Root vegetables:

Asparagus	Avocado
Artichoke hearts	Carrots
Brussels sprouts	Spinach
Broccoli	Zucchini
Celery	Cabbage

Cauliflower	Eggplant
Green Onions	Peppers (All Kinds)
Parsley	Coconut oil

Contrary to popular belief, fats in food don't make you overweight – carbohydrates do and the typical American food has a lot of them. Natural oils and body fats are your body's desired method of producing energy so it's important to provide your body with what it's requesting! Below are some of the greatest kinds of foods that contain paleo oils and fats that you can provide your body with needed sustained energy.

Paleo Diet Nuts

Our favorite nuts! (Does that sound bad?) Nuts are definitely Paleo. Be wary though as cashews are full of fat and so delicious that it can be easy to eat a whole jar in one meeting. If you're trying to lose weight, limit the serving of nuts you are allowed and stick to it!

You can also try a decent pecan/walnut/ almond nut mix as well. The following chart shows some of the good Paleo Diet nuts:

Almonds	Cashews
Hazelnuts	Pecans
Pine Nuts	Paleo Diet Fruits
Pumpkin Seeds	Sunflower Seeds
Macadamia Nut	Walnuts

Paleo Diet fruits

Paleo Diet fruits are not only attractive but also they are very good for you. Paleo accepted fruits are those that contain great quantities of fructose that is much more preferred over HFCS (high-fructose corn syrup) – but it is still sugar. If you're looking to lose extra weight on the Paleo Diet, you'll need to limit the fruits and focus more on the root vegetables allowed on the Paleo diet. However, feel free to enjoy 1-3 portions of fruit a day. Check out this list of Paleo Diet fruits and see if you're not starving by the time you get to the bottom! (We'll admit, we're partial to the blackberries).

Apple	Avocado
Blackberries	Papaya
Peaches	Plums
Mango	Blueberries
Lychee	Figs
Grapes	Lemon
Strawberries	Watermelon

Oranges	Bananas
Raspberries	Cantaloupe
Tangerine	Pineapple

List of Foods Not Acceptable on the Paleo Diet

This is an essential list of food that is not acceptable on the Paleo Diet. It's very difficult to let these types of foods go once you start out on your Paleo food journey, but as you continue you will find that it gets easier and you will discover many Paleo food alternatives to replace your old favorites. The first few weeks will be hard, but if you make the switch, it'll be very beneficial to you. We have the ability. Here's the final list of foods that are not acceptable on the Paleo Diet.

- No fast food
(candy, , ice cream ,crackers, snack foods)

- No Beans
  (lima beans, dark beans, peanuts, baked beans)

- No Sugar or Synthetic Sugar
  (Splenda, pure cane, corn syrup, honey, maltodextrin, Equal, Stevia, agave nectar, syrup, etc.)

- No Starches
  (wheat goods, corn goods, pasta, cereals, rice, oatmeal, bread)

- No Dairy

- No Alcohol

Chapter 4   Paleo exercise

In modern life, we use lots of instruments and machines for exercise to keep our body fit and to make body muscles. But it is possible to make a fit body and impressive muscles just with some movements called paleo exercise. This is the type of movements that the ancient cavemen did perform to survive against adverse and unpredictable environment and to protect themselves from wild animals. There are several steps of paleo exercise. They are discussed below:

1. Warm-up: Before starting any exercise, you need to warm up your body muscles. Otherwise, muscles can be injured during exercise. For this, you can use a treadmill or simply can walk or run for several minutes, can jump, and do some movements of every part of the body.

2. Squatting: Squatting is the bending of the knee and hips keeping the back straight. You can take some weight on your shoulder and hold the weight when squatting but it is not very much necessary. You can also perform simple squatting without any weight.

3. Bending: You'll have to hold tow, simple weights in your two hands and bend side to side. At least 10 times bending is needed in each side.

4. Lunging: Take a barbell on your shoulder, then step up on a chair or bench alternating the legs in every step. Do at least 20 times.

5. Pushing: Stand up and hold a cable or elastic band. Then push forward like punching. Do it 20 times with each arm. Switch the arm and repeat it.

6. Pulling: Just do the reverse movement of pushing. Hold the cable or elastic band and pull it down instead of pushing.

7. Twisting: Now hold the cable with both arms, keep the arms straight and twist in both sides. Do it 10 times in each side.

8. Lifting weight: Lift any heavy things. It can be anything like rock, tree, tires or can use dumbbell and barbell. When you lift any weight from the ground, there is a possibility to injure the veins of waist. So, be careful

about this or use waistband when lifting any
heavy weight.

9. Dips or pushup: Dips is a very useful
Paleo exercise which affects on chest,
shoulder, back and arms. No additional
weight is required for dips. Just use the body
weight. Pushup or dips is raising lowering the
body, placing two hands on the ground.

10. Resting: In all exercise programs, resting
is a most necessary thing. Our body muscles
need rest to make the proper development
and to maintain fitness. So, it is generally
advised to do exercise in every alternative day.

Also, it is to mention that during exercise, it is
needed to drink a lot of water because during
exercise, our body temperature becomes high
and water controls the temperature inside. So,
after completing each set of exercise, drinking
water is must.

The basic goal of paleo exercise is to improve
body strength and fitness. Paleo diet is also
helpful to keep the fitness during paleo
workout.

Chapter 5   Top Paleo habits

Human beings are creatures of habit. Most things you do on a daily basis, you do automatically. Our brain tends to create habits so we can focus on the things in our life that really matter. For example, when you are driving a car you are doing this effortlessly (most of the time). You are not thinking about all the little steps you are taking. You just step into your car, turn on the engine, and go. And all this while talking with the person next to you. Why is that? This is because we created this habit by repeating it often. If you had to think consciously about every little step you needed to take, you wouldn't be able to focus on other things.

The same thing goes with your diet. Most of the time, we eat the same thing, the same amount, and at the same time every day. This helps us to focus on the important tasks in our life and not on our food.

Replace Your Food One Step at a Time

When you want to implement the Paleo Diet, it is very important to do this one step at a time. It is too difficult to change your whole diet overnight. You can try it, but most of the time, you will fall back because it's too much to digest at once. It's like the saying eat the elephant piece by piece'. It is important to replace your bad foods with good foods. Here is a 5-step action plan for how to implement the Paleo Diet immediately.

1.Start with the beverages

The easiest and most important thing you can change overnight is replacing all your beverages with water and green tea. A lot of the daily sodas and juices we consume contain a lot of added sugars, toxins, and empty calories. The best thing you can do is to avoid these beverages and consume water or green tea instead.You will notice that you are going to feel much better because you are getting rid of all of those artificial drinks. If you really don't like the taste of plain water or green tea, you can be creative with it. Start mixing water with fresh fruit. This will give you the sweet taste while drinking a lot of water.

2.Replace Sugar with Honey

Honey is Paleo, sweet and a lot healthier than sugar. So, if you really have a sweet tooth and can't possibly find a way to get rid of sweets, I highly recommend that you replace your sugar with honey.

3.Replace the Bad Carbohydrates with Paleo Substitutes

Some of the toughest things to remove from our diet are processed carbs. I always loved potatoes, pastas, and bread. We ate these things a lot at home and when I started to change my diet, I couldn't find a way to get rid of these carbs. I tried to eat more vegetables, but it did not do the trick for me. The one thing that helped me to control my carb cravings were Paleo substitutes. Paleo substitutes taste just like your favorite carbs, but are healthy and Paleo.

4.Start Eating Grass-Fed Meat, Fish, and Eggs

If you didn't already, start eating grass fed meat, fish, and eggs. You can choose which meats, fish, or eggs you'll eat, but it is important to eat them all in a good balance. The best way to implement this is by trying a new meat, fish, and egg every day and writing down which ones you really like. Fine-tune this until you have a perfect mix you like

5.Only Keep Paleo Foods at Home

Start throwing away (or giving away if you think throwing away food is a waste) all the non-Paleo foods. Also, start buying Paleo foods only. This will help you stick with the diet when you are having a hard time. When you start to implement the Paleo Diet, it will come as a willpower challenge to stay away from pastas, bread, or other things you really love. If you keep them at home, you will most likely eat them, even if you weren't intending to eat them at first. So get rid of these foods.

Chapter 6   Paleo and Weight Loss

Here are a number of great tips of how to lose weight on the Paleo diet:

1. Keep your diet simple.

One of the reasons the Paleo diet is so helpful with weight loss is due to its ability to help you decrease the number of calories that you consume unknowingly. Studies have demonstrated that eating smaller portions leads to consuming less food, which in turn helps you to avoid having an excess of calories.

2. Be sure to eat enough.

Numerous Paleo newbies think that less food is always better when it comes to losing weight. This belief causes you to deprive your body of the calories and nutrients needed to be at your best and reasons further pressure. Lessening your caloric intake lowers your latent metabolic rate, which can cause you to actually gain weight. No matter what diet you choose, starving yourself should never be an option. Calories are a vital part of our existence.

3. Eat enough carbs to provide for your activity level.

Carbohydrate intake is completely different, and I've seen people who do fairly well on a low carb diet, while others crash and burn. Typically, the main issue is the quantity and level of activity the person is involved in, as many of my patients trying to lose weight are taking part in challenging strength exercise machines, such as Crossfit, or spend many hours at the local fitness center.

4. Change throughout the day.

Being too inactive can decrease the benefits of your exercise program and prevent weight loss. If you work in an office, travel by car and watch too many hours of television at night, it's not hard to understand how you could spend a large portion of your waking hours sitting on your bottom. Also, a workout alone isn't enough to counteract the damaging effects of a sedentary lifestyle. When it comes to weight loss, having energy throughout the whole day, and not just during the 60 minutes you work at the gymnasium, is a vital part of a healthy routine.

5. Never do it by yourself.

One of the toughest parts of losing weight is trying to do it all by yourself. Creating major life changes without any help from friends is not only difficult, but often unmanageable. Asking friends or family to inspire you, or even make changes along with you, can significantly increase your achievement in any major life change, specifically the change to a Paleo diet. You can share plans, arrange partner challenges, and inspire each other on your trip to good health.

6. Discourse your entire life, not just food and application.

Focus on managing stress using mind-body methods, like meditation or yoga. Think about using shopping and meal plans to help you decrease the stress that comes along with starting a big life change. Spend time with friends and family, and gather support in your weight loss efforts. You'll be more likely to lose weight and keep it off for the long haul. And you'll really be able to enjoy living your life.

The Positive weight loss isn't about the number of calories in your low-carb tortillas, or "counteracting" each treat with an hour of sweating it out at the gym. Striving to starve your body into shape without considering your natural metabolic challenges and food desires will be unsuccessful and will not bring the desired results. The way to permanent weight loss is mending the harm brought to your metabolism and hormonal systems from the toxic modern food environment; a ketogenic Paleo diet gives your body the opportunity to heal itself, making a solid foundation for your lasting fitness, not a temporary change to your tie size.

Conclusion

Thank you again for downloading this book!

I hope this book was able to help you to know about Paleo Diet.

Finally, if you enjoyed this book, then I'd like to ask you for a favor, would you be kind enough to leave a review for this book on Amazon? It'd be greatly appreciated!

Thank you and good luck!

Book 2

Essential oils

A quick beginner guide

By Rick Paul

Table of Contents

Introduction

I want to thank you and congratulate you for downloading the book, Essential oils.

This book contains proven steps and strategies on how to use Essential oils.

For hundreds of years, essential oils have been used to for various medicinal purposes and lucky for you, they are still here to make your life healthy and awesome. Essential oils are known to combat stress, improve the quality of sleep, fight flu and cold, increase concentration, rid the body of toxins, aid in reducing muscle spasms and reduce chronic pains. Additionally, they are used for cleaning purposes. For instance, Lavender is normally recommended for to relieving stress, banish insomnia and improve the general concentration.

When cooling the skin during hot days is necessary, peppermint essential oil will be handy. Below is an introduction to essential oils on how to use them and why they are the best choice.

Essential oils are hydroponic liquids that are extracted from particular plants and when diluted into the right concentration have healing properties. In recent years essential oils have made their way back into society after having been overlooked for years, mainly due to the modern chemical medicine.

I hope that I have succeeded in making a book that not only is incredibly informative, but also accessible for those who might not have a lot of experience using essential oils.

If you are new to essential oils, you have found the right place. With just a little effort, you will open up an entirely new world of natural solutions to you.

Let's get started!

Chapter 1   What is Essential oils

Essential oils usually are extracted from flowers and also plants, they've been used for many centuries nevertheless remain as valuable things for aromatherapy and also traditional medicinal systems.

There are many of vital oils accessible nowadays, the commonest ones are usually are numbered from 90. An increasing number of are produced so that you can treat illnesses like melanoma, HIV signs and symptoms, asthma, heart strokes along with bronchitis. Essential oils tend to be used with regard to relaxation and massage purposes, but the uses aren't limited.

There are a variety of particular person benefits with regards to the essential oil that is certainly being used as well as the effect from the essential oil depends on where it got their start in.

Why Essential Oils?

It truly is cheaper to work with essential natural oils for household cleaning as compared to using professional cleaning solutions. The essential oils may also be anti-viral, antibacterial, anti-microbial and anti-fungal. They are exceptionally uncomplicated and 100% safe for work with by people coming from all ages and professions.

Essential oils are certainly not only enjoyable and simple to operate, but additionally they work; many people never fail. A few days of employing this products and you're sure of reaping this benefits. Unlike numerous products available on the market that are full of toxins, essential natural oils are non-toxic hence there're safe for the body, the children and actually the pets are certainly not harmed. Of likewise great significance about the use of essential natural oils is they are eco-friendly; at any given time when ecological deterioration worries are therefore high, this is the ideal solution. The extent through which essential oils help the human physical and mental well being is merely remarkable; there're the best substitute for our tribulations.

How to use essential oils.

Just before we commence the talk, it ought to be noted which essential oils usually are not allowed to be directly put on one's skin. In order to become safe, it is strongly recommended that the main oils are generally first diluted. The first task, though, is to test that your skin are not harshly troubled by the fat by assessment it first. This is normally done by simply placing the drop in the oil mixture over a small swatch of the skin. You should leave this particular drop of fat on your skin for at the least 24 hours in order to make certain that you don't have any harmful kind of reaction.

Make sure you include vital oils as part of your daily baths ritual; 8-10 drops added in the bathing water is sufficient to rid the entire body of just about any stress. Lavender, frankincense, roman chamomile, grapefruit in addition to jasmine ought to be in your collection regarding bath moment essential natural skin oils. After a great work out and about, eucalyptus vital oils will likely be great intended for relaxing the muscles in addition to reducing joint pains.

Inhaling vital oils will take your latest mood and provides it a great unimaginable lift up. Experience the magic regarding essential oils in your mood by simply putting 5 in order to 10 drops of the favorite fat in sizzling water. Inhale the steam severally having a towel protected over your brain. Another way to get this done is to put at least 5 drops in the essential oil as part of your dehumidifier; fill your home with fantastic fragrance in addition to relax. For any great goodnight rest, a few drops while on an essential oil around the pillow will work.

How are essential oils extracted?

Essential oils may be extracted while using the distillation method. One process could possibly be steam distillation, the vapor will move upwards over the plant materials causing small oil sacs to be able to rapture and also release their own vapor. Following the oil continues to be extracted, the steam will be combined and cooled and would be condensed. It's going to be separated after which filtered. In addition, there are other processes to have essential natural skin oils like hydro- distillation where inside plant material will likely be boiled in water; this process could be used for flowers.

Why are essential oils effective?

Essential oils carry the ability to protect humans against disease-causing microbes. Many essential oils have been proven to be stimulants or sedatives for humans. The plants were able to adapt to the growing needs of insects and humans, and the essential oil constituents is a proof of this evolution in plants. Human bodies have been biologically programmed to respond to the components of the oils through the receptor sites of the body, the neurochemicals as well as the enzymes that contribute to the benefits of the essential oils.

What essential oils are considered therapeutic?

Tea tree is one good example of an essential oil that can be used to cure a number of illnesses. It can be used for muscle aches and pains and can relieve people from migraine. Other therapeutic oils that can be used for healing will include citrus oils and olive oil.

Chapter 2 Introducing Aromatherapies

Aromatherapy is a kind of alternative medicine, mainly based on essential oils and additional aromatic plant compounds to enhance health as well as mood of the individual. It is also popularly known as Essential Oil Therapy.

Why do People Go after Aromatherapy?

Aromatherapy is totally chemical free and supplement based remedy. Using essential oils within aromatherapy keeps your environment,air pollution free mainly because those essential oils would be the extracts connected with pure herbal products collected in the nature.

For countless years people have put their rely upon several types of essential oils for their therapeutic gains.There will vary ways connected with applying essential oils for aromatherapy with respect to the goals you may need to achieve.

Massage is often a commonly used way of the distribution of aromatherapy gains using essential oils. The rubbing down if done properly by way of a professional counselor can best target the right muscles for optimal gains. But any other person can certainly still find out the art and achieve accomplishment in relaxing tensions along with relieving nervousness. Whether essential oils penetrate the skin or to never achieve any health improvements remains extremely debatable. For many years Aromatherapists claimed that may be how the particular oils treated, but modern-day scientific testing points to the truth that the benefits have been realized by way of inhalation.

Essential Oils for Your Family

Essential oils would be the intense essence of place material, mostly employed in aromatherapy. They may be entirely prepared from botanical matter. They may be mostly confused with all the synthetic perfume oils, which might be chemical regeneration associated with scents prepared mainly via coal tar. Even when the scent of perfume oils could possibly be identical to essential skin oils, they don't get similar element structure and as a consequence, they won't get a similar treatment effect.In fact,the using synthetic perfume oils is restricted to perfumery. Children aromatherapy is a kind of aromatherapy intended to assist throughout, improving the particular happiness and also wellness associated with children.

How to introduce aromatherapy to children

Place 2-3 drops of essential oil on a piece of tissue and keep it close when feeding her or him. This will make the child associate the aroma with comfort and love. You can use this scent during the night to assist the child sleep. When a child is left in a sitter in the presence of aroma, it reassures and comfort her or him.

Use of essential oils in cleaning of children

Children ones like bathtub water, which has a good scent. Roman chamomile and lavender are good selections for youngsters. Use 2-3 drops divorce lawyers Atlanta bath. Citrus oil can be employed as a cleaning agent in the home. Just include few declines of fruit, orange, mandarin or even bergamot fat to drinking water, moisten a sheet of cloth with all the mixture and wipe the children's rooms. Scent the children's drawers keeping the night moment clothing with oil solution put on cotton golf balls. It will deliver the youngsters a sweet dream.

Dosage of essential oil for children

Children respond very well to low dosage of essential oil particularly for irritability and anger. Use a third of adult dosage because their skin is delicate. When adding essential oils to bath water, shake well before blending the correct number of drops with water. Only use those oils safe for children.

Different kinds of Aromatherapy Oils that one should keep at hand

Lavender: It offers a wonderful outside pleasing experiencing. It is often a floral cologne with touch of sweet taste. With calming effect this works question to relax the violent mind. Medicinally, it relieves pain and also minor wounds along with insect hits.

Peppermint: Due to it's one of the main constituents "menthol" it has icy sensation that arouse mental sharpness of the users. Not only that, it sooths migraine, headache, painful muscles, and above all problem of digestion.

Eucalyptus: It is a clean and fresh aroma to open up your congested airways. It is an antibacterial, antimicrobial, antifungal as well as antiinflammatory. It works wonder for asthma, cough and cold, and congestion.

Lemon: It helps to remove bad aura and boost mental alertness. As an antifungal it is wonderful for fixing cuts, cuts, and several other minor injuries. For clearing the air passage, rubbing it on throat and chest will give instant relief.

Tea Tree:. It's famous instead medicine. The astringent on the oil relieves oily secretions over the surface of the skin. The terpinen on the oil soothes little injuries. Contain a little cost you shampoo intended for super cleaning of your respective scalp. Using crucial oils inside aromatherapy may be the latest addition towards cosmetic therapy.

Chapter 3 How does Aromatherapy work

Different ways of uses and applications

Different ways of using essential oils for aromatherapy are widely accepted and many of them optimize inhalation. Depending on the method of application and intended goals, the essential oils are added in just a few drops not exceeding 10% of an ounce (600 drops) of the carrier oil to which they are added. The following are the main categories of uses of different essential oils for different therapeutic method and how they work.

For Skincare

A blend of facial oil can be created by adding up to 15 drops of an essential oil to a carrier oil of choice, unscented lotion or cream. Rosemary is one of the essential oils that can be added to a skin cream to help in rewinding the aging clock. Facial steam for skincare and cleansing routines requires about 5 drops added in a facial steam or a pint of water that is warm. 5 drops of a favorite essential oil can be added to honey, egg white, moistened clay or mashed avocado, for facial masks. For the entire body use, add 3 drops of an essential oil like pink grapefruit that can simulate to the bristles of a bath brush. You can brush from your toes or fingers towards the heart to experience the stimulating effect.

For treatment

Inhalation is probably the best ways involving using essential natural oils for treatment involving problems like sinus or bronchial illnesses. You can add about drops for you to steaming water in a bowl. You are able to capture the steam by using a towel for inhaling while your sight remain closed before the oil smell diminishes. The procedure is usually repeated every 5 hrs if necessary. Up to 9 fat drops can also be added to a humidifier's water after which left running immediately. A nebulizer via microdiffusion produces micro-particles of your essential in their particular millions to optimize the effect of inhalation regarding treatment. Adding gas drops to normal water in bath tubs, Jacuzzi, showers and for easy use in topical applications is additionally meant for treatment of numerous ailments.

For household uses

When cleaning different surfaces around the house, essential oils can be used with various detergents and soaps. They will leave behind their fragrances and continue to provide the benefits of aromatherapy for hours. They can be used when doing laundry, washing dishes, flavoring and general cleaning.

How Essential Oils Work to Relieve the Patients?

Aromatic or Essential oils stimulate the olfactory nerves from the patients along with send signals for the Neuro-receptors in your brain. It is a result of this reason that after you employ them a good electro-chemical answer is induced that promotes the total amount in your nervous process and aid relieving hassles. Though there are many of man-made aromatic oils you can buy that amount to less. Yet, these oils aren't recommended. For top results, use certified crucial oils which can be free by pesticides.

Do fragrant healing soy candles truly work?

All over again, fragrant healing may be utilized by individuals everywhere internationally since the starting of development. It might become tricky to contend against the viability of the practice regardless to the fact that its belongings have been totally psychosomatic. Inside correlation, western medication offers just barely did start to understand the adequacy or maybe fragrance based treatment.

Fragrance based treatment utilizes the inbuilt mending forces of the pith or stench of specific plant life, blooms, roots, etc. A standard lighting scented with counterfeit aroma won't have the same effect. The explanation behind it is on the reasons that fundamental herbal oils are inferred from common sources although consistently scented luminous made of wax utilizes chemicals in order to copy certain fragrances. The body is aware of which aroma can be common and that fragrance is constructed.

When you light a typical scented candle, you merely about quickly start to smell the perfume being discharged because of the scent or aroma that may be imbued with the flame wax. In the event you are useful to the solid, impactful aromas connected with current scented candle lights, it may take that you while to stench the fragrance being discharged with a fragrant healing soy luminous made of wax.

The contrasts involving a fragrance misleadingly processed by an aroma along with a smell regularly earned by and critical oil are considerable. Scent fragrances are generally helpful in that they can trigger memory receptors as well as subsequently influence tendency. Nonetheless, crucial oils handle this level and a noticeably much deeper degree. It is not so much the aroma from the key oil that may be helpful. It happens to be accepted that the chemicals in these oils possess a measurable impact within the physical body.

It's always best to utilize soy wax when making use of key plant oils for a few reasons. Firstly, it blazes neatly and doesn't antagonistically influence the scent of the crucial oils. It likewise blazes cooler, which permits the scent being scattered even more gradually and even more equally, in supplement, the oils aren't warmed up to the point where the critical oils are damaged. This can take place with paraffin given it smolders sultrier as well as producing carbon based sediment when blazed.

On the point when using a fragrant healing soy luminous made of wax, it is prescribed that you simply discover a relaxed spot to sit and breathe in the fragrance for no less than a half hr. This will supply the vital oils time to communicate using your body.

The general uses of Aromatherapy

Aromatherapy is used generally for flu, colds, sore muscles, relaxation etc.

Bath: If you use this therapy for bathing, then fill the tub and add essential oils. In addition, to take a small cup of milk and add the oils with a tablespoon of honey and then add it into the water.

Shower: After a shower, take five to seven drops of essential oils on a damp, clean cloth and then rub it on the whole body. After that, allow it to dry in the air.

Compress: This therapy is excellent for lessening the pain. This oil is useful for menstrual cramps or strained muscles, etc. Add four to seven drops of Essential Oil into a bowl of water. Take a cloth, dip it into the water and wring it out. Now place the cloth on the painful area. Repeat it, when the cloth cools. A plastic sheet or towel can be covered on the warm cloth. It will help to keep the warm for long time. This therapy is very much helpful for getting relief from menstrual cramps.

Jacuzzi: If you go after bath tub or Jacuzzi, then add 3 drops of essential oil for an individual. You can repeat it after every 30 minutes. But remember that a few essential oil can damage the plastic tub.

Bath salts: Take some Epsom salts, baking soda and sea salt and mix them well. Then add six to ten drops essential oil with this mixture and blend it well. You can add it with warm water for bathe or can rub this blend before the bath.It helps to cure aching muscle or sore.

Chapter 4 List of common oils and their uses

Here are some of the essential oils used for weight loss:

Grapefruit Oil:

Grapefruit oil naturally suppresses the appetite through a process known as lipolysis. It also dissolves fats. It combines very well with lavender in a Whiffer aromatherapy pendant.

Peppermint Oil:

Peppermint oil helps one to feel fuller. It actually affects the part of the brain that deals with satiety or feeling full. Dr. Alan Hirsch of the Smell and Taste Treatment and Research Institute of Chicago recommends that inhaling the aroma of these essential oils throughout the day and before each meal can greatly help to curb appetite.

Tangerine Oil:

Tangerine essential oil is another citrus-based oil that may help with weight loss. It also helps to regulate metabolism, create a feeling of happiness and reduce anxiety. However, one should not go out in the sun after applying tangerine oil. It is often combined with bergamot or lavender.

Vanilla Oil:

Vanilla essential oils might help curb the desire for food for sweets which can be very common throughout women. They can be used in a diffuser or maybe in aromatherapy candles to aid curb cravings. Reducing the volume of sweets in one's diet regime can go a considerable ways towards significant weight loss and reducing the danger of diabetes.

Bergamot Oil:

Bergamot oil doesn't directly curb hunger but has soothing effects within the mind. It basically eliminates stress and creates an awareness of of well-being. Dr. Hirsch recommends that bergamot could be combined with lavender oil which has calming properties. Owing to the truth that people tend to consume more when there're stressed, smelling bergamot oil can establish a sense connected with calmness that continues them from eating once they are not truly hungry.

Patchouli Oil:

Patchouli essential oil can help to effectively control appetite. It can also be used as a sedative and relaxation aid. These oils can be used in a bath or in a diffuser. When used in a bath, 10 -15 drops of the oil should be added to the bath water. Patchouli works more effectively in the evening hours. When used in a diffuser, the same amount should be added to an oil diffuser and inhaled deeply.

Rose Geranium Oil:

Rose geranium is a very powerful essential oil with mood lifting qualities. It therefore reduces appetite which results in one eating less food.

Ylang ylang Oil:

Used to clarify thoughts and assist in a feeling of wellness and calm. It therefore curbs appetite resulting to consumption of less food.

Dill Oil

This oil is extracted from dill seeds and has sedative properties. It does not contain cholesterol and low in calories. It therefore effectively contributes to weight loss.

Orange Oil:

Helps overcome depression and gives emotional support.

Essential oils will help in weight-loss through which affects one's disposition. Depression and stress tend to be the reasons behind overeating. Using the calming vital oils such as lavender regarding massage and bath will help relax the entire body, improve your mood therefore eliminate some of the psychological causes for overeating.

Here are the essential oils used for a quick relieve from headaches:

Lavender Oil:

Lavender oil is probably the most well-liked and low-priced essential herbal oils for head ache relieve out there. It incorporates a high percent of esters and hence it provides anti-inflammatory and also sedative components.

It encourages relation, helps someone to sleep and also treats headaches and depression symptoms. Lavender oil works better when employed to alleviate headaches at night time hours.

Jasmine Oil:

Though it's a bit more expensive than other essential oils, Jasmine oil has therapeutic properties that are very strong hence making it very valuable. This oil provides energy and calms emotions at the same time. It also improves the tone of a person's skin. A wide range of Sandalwood, Bergamot, Rose and citrus oils can be blended with Jasmine very effectively.

Chamomile Oil:

Both Roman and German Chamomile oil have powerful properties that can be used to treat premenstrual syndrome which is a major cause of headache. Chamomile has also been recommended by health practitioners to calm severe headache resulting from irritability. It can be blended in massage oil or a few drops can be placed in a bath, vaporizer or diffuser.When combined with creams and lotions, Chamomile becomes more efficient for headache relieve.

Rose Oil:

Just like Jasmine, Rose is a multipurpose fat. It's normally blended with other crucial oils such as Bergamot, patchouli, cedarwood, chamomile and also sandalwood. It can be utilized for anti-depressant to generate feelings associated with calmness. Since trauma is a common reason for severe headaches, this oil can promote over emotional healing on this condition. Rose oil for headaches may be added in order to massage fat or bath tub product.

Eucalyptus oil:

Eucalyptus radiata and Eucalyptus globules contain a significant amount of oxide 1, 8-Cineole. 1, 8-Cineole acts as both an expectorant as well as an antiinflammatory. Eucalyptus oil helps to ease headaches especially those associated with sinus headaches.

Taking Care of Your Skin with Essential Oils

Tea Tree Oil

Tea tree oil is usually an alternate prestigious oil around the grounds it has outstanding medicinal components, for illustration, antibacterial, antiviral, antifungal, germicide and also pain reduce. Thusly they have the beautiful abilities to extract, clean, and also sooth chafed, aroused skin conditions. It is actually quick acting and may clear way up skin inflammation, flaws and also pimples rapidly.

Sandalwood oil

Sandalwood should be to a fantastic degree saturating oil that is certainly useful to get dried out or dried out skin. Sandalwood may evacuate lines and wrinkles, scars, in addition to almost minimal differences. It truly is likewise a antibacterial in addition to antifungal which often can lessen the wedding of pimple inflammation in addition to skin ailments.

Lemon oil

Lemon oil and different citrus oils are extraordinary for clearing up pimple inflammation quick by evacuating the abundance sebum and oil on the face. It has extraordinary recuperating and remedial qualities particularly when connected to healthy skin. Lemon oil can light up ones composition by evacuating dead skin cells. Be that as it may, it can result in skin staining when laid open to steer daylight, accordingly it's basic to stay out of the sun instantly in the wake of applying lemon oil.

Clary Sage Oil

Clary sage is advantageous for skin conditions are produced by hormone lopsided attributes, for illustration, pimple infection, wrinkles along with barely incomparable differences. Clary Sage has a comparative structure to human being hormones coupled these lines maybe it's utilized to be able to supplement with regard to imbalanced bodily hormones when uncovered into the body. It furthermore goes about being an antibacterial along with astringent to be able to murder contamination along with purge acute wounds.

Myrrh Oil

Myrrh oil has been utilized for a long time and within aged times utilized as a part of an emollient to treat just about any illness. It has been known to treat dry skin, wrinkles, rashes, imperfections, dermatitis, and microscopic organisms in the skin.

Natural Essential Oil Based Hair Care Products

List of Essential Oils

Lavender Oil: it has proven hair benefits and works well for all hair types. Lavender oil is a good treatment for itching and dandruff and it is helpful in improving hair growth and controlling hair breakage.

Chamomile Oil: is known to soothe the hair and scalp, and helps to retract inflamed skin cells, to alleviate dandruff conditions and itching scaly scalp.

Peppermint Oil: helps to nourish the hair by stimulating blood flow to the hair root.

Rosemary Oil: is useful for flaky itchy scalp and dandruff problems.

Tea Tree Oil: it helps to keep the scalp free of fungal problems and bacteria and it is a great moisturizer for the hair.

Lemon Oil: is beneficial for oily hair and it is recommended for dandruff and lice.

Myrrh Oil: is very good for dry hair and dandruff.

Carrier Oils

Carrier oils are another type of oils for hair that can help carry the essential oil onto the skin. They are derived from nuts or seeds by maceration or cold pressing. Carrier oils are nourishing the hair and they are great moisturizers and strengtheners.

Oils for Normal Hair

These essential oils are working best for normal hair:

• Clary Sage

• Rosemary

• Cedar wood

• Thyme

• Lemon

• Lavender

• Geranium

The best carrier oils to use for normal hair are almond, jojoba, and borage.

Chapter 5   Recipe

Recipe for Skin Moisturizing Lotion

This recipe is essentially for a great skin moisturizing lotion for everybody:

Ingredients

- 15 drops of natural Geranium

- 8 lotion base ounces

- 5 drops of ylang ylang

- 10 drops of some myrrh

Procedure

Before you start to make your skin layer care blend, it is significant to note that you ought to always use therapeutically pure grade essential oils. The procedure is simply adding essential oils into a lotion in addition to mixing the mixture lightly. Add the label that contains the substances you utilised in the box.

Myrrh in addition to geranium usually are some typical essential oils which have been used extensively to heal your skin. Adding ylang ylang will simply improve the oils fragrance, which is often a very recipe will cool in addition to soften skin and have tried them in cleaning some unsightly stains from hands and wrists. key theory to aromatherapy regarding consumers. If customers do not like the aroma they will also steer clear of buying the goods. This is simply an illustration of this what you can use, there vary combinations offered.

For skins which have been so dried up, it is significant to increase 10 declines of Roman Chamomile, Rose and Sandalwood in order to one's 8 oz of bottom lotion. Be sure only pure therapeutic essential grade natural oils are largely used.

If an example may be so much thinking about making their very own lotion make use of by introducing some essential oils, then this old recipe will cool in addition to soften skin and have tried them in cleaning some unsightly stains from hands and wrists.

Ingredients

- 1 ounce freshly squeezed lemon juice
- 1 ounce of rosewater
- 10 therapeutic grade essential oils of choice
- 1 ounce of glycerin

Procedure

Put all this items in a clean bottle and shake them gently. Label the bottle with some instructions of shaking well before any use and label all the ingredients used on the outside of the bottle, and then store them in a clean refrigerator. This mixture needs to be used for a maximum of three weeks, hence, require one to use them in small amounts at one particular time.

Recipe for a Winter Lotion

Ingredients

- Half a cup of rose water or distilled water

- 1 tablespoonful of lecithin

- Half a cup of jojoba oil

- 1 vitamin E capsule

- 15 drops of one's favorite essential oils therapeutic grade

Procedure

Put all the products not including vitamins At the capsule inside a blender as well as whip these people until these people form a fine nice cream. Feel liberated to add more distilled water when you really need a slimmer lotion. Add oil and e vitamin capsule at the end of it. Lecithin is often a mixing agent that aids water as well as oil adhere together. Mix them all well as store these people in quite clean storage units labeled along with ingredients utilized.

Cream oil is often a particular vegetable oil that's some water put into it. This particular however, is an ideal skin color moisturizer.Cream is thicker as compared to lotion oil mainly because it has much less water. The persistence of almost any lotion helps make the lotion suited to oily or perhaps normal skin color. Cream has the spreading easiness for the skin and does not leave greasy coats onto it. Adding vital oils for you to skin will certainly enhance making use of essential natural skin oils for skin care therapeutic benefit.

Conclusion

Thank you again for downloading this book!

I hope this book was able to help you to know about Essential oils.

Finally, if you enjoyed this book, then I'd like to ask you for a favor, would you be kind enough to leave a review for this book on Amazon? It'd be greatly appreciated!

Thank you and good luck!

Preview Of 'Alcoholism Addiction by Rick Paul

You may not realize it at first, but when your sips of wine or vodka happens too often, such as when you drink even if you are eating lunch, or you have become accustomed to drinking whenever you have problems, that may already be trouble. People oftentimes realize that they are addicted to alcohol when it is already too late.

Alcoholism is a chronic and often progressive disease that includes problems controlling your drinking, being preoccupied with alcohol, continuing to use alcohol even when it causes problems, having to drink more to get the same effect (physical dependence),or having withdrawal symptoms when you rapidly decrease or stop drinking.

Many millions of people can take alcohol or they can leave it - they can drink normally, enjoying an occasional glass of wine, or a drink with a meal or on a special occasion. That type of drinking is certainly permitted by the Bible. Alcohol used to mask chronic symptoms of anxiety, depression, interpersonal issues, family or work problems and other issues can quickly and decisively lead to a progressive emotional, physical and spiritual condition where things will go badly in a hurry.

Alcohol can be an uncomfortable subject. If you have an alcohol problem it's not easy to admit it and seek help. If you know someone with a problem, confronting them with the issue or knowing how to help can be very difficult. If this describes you, it will take a bit of courage, but please keep reading. Set denial aside for a moment and you'll see, there is real hope.

You will get exact and reliable information in regards to the topic and issue covered. The book is sold with the information that the publisher is not necessary to render accounting, officially acceptable, or otherwise, professional services. If information is necessary, legal or acceptable, an experienced individual in the profession should be ordered..